The Guide to Everyday Healing and Calm

Mindful reflections and gentle rituals to help you rediscover calm and come home to yourself.

Dedication Page

For the ones who hold everything inside, stay strong for others, and quietly rebuild themselves when no one sees their effort.

For those who worry they are falling behind — you were never off track, only finding your way back to yourself.

And for every deep-feeler who heals slowly and doubts their own strength — you are not broken, you are becoming.

© 2025 S. Shelly

Published by Stardust Press

All rights reserved.

No part of this publication may be reproduced, distributed, or transmitted in any form or by any means, including photocopying, recording, or other electronic or mechanical methods, without the prior written permission of the publisher, except in the case of brief quotations embodied in critical reviews and certain other non-commercial uses permitted by copyright law.

ISBN: 978-1-9193876-6-6

First Edition

Printed and distributed worldwide by IngramSpark.

Contents

🌿 Part One – The Space Around You

• The Foot Bath for Grounding & Release	11
• Grounding – Returning to the Earth	14
• Seasonal Energy – Living in Flow with Nature	20
• A Breath of Fresh Air – For You & Your Home	26
• Cleansing with Sage & Sacred Smoke	28
• The Power of Salt Lamps & Real Plants	31
• Feng Shui Flow – Inviting Harmony into Your Home	34
• Aromatherapy & Candles – Lighting Your Intention	37

💧 Part Two – The Body You Live In

• Hydration & Natural Detox	42
• Vitamins, Minerals & Cyclical Balance	45
• Reflexology – Touchpoints for Calm	48
• Gentle Self-Massage & Body Awareness	51

- Sleep, Rest & the Art of Stillness   54

🔥 Part Three – The Energy Within

- Crystals & Their Healing Frequencies   59
- Developing Intuitive Awareness   62
- Chakra Balancing & Cleansing Meditation   65
- Journaling as Energy Release   71

🌱 Part Four – Bringing It Together

- Building Daily & Weekly Routines   78
- Moments of Light – Daily Reflections for Calm   83
- Gratitude, Faith & Trusting the Process   89
- Your Personal Resilience Kit   95
- Leaving Work Behind & Coming Home to Yourself   102

Epilogue – The Light You Carry Forward

Introduction

There comes a point in every busy life when the pace begins to feel unsustainable and the mind asks for a pause.

This guide was created for those moments — a space to slow down, to breathe, and to reconnect with what keeps you balanced.

Inside these pages you'll find simple, practical ways to support your wellbeing: small daily rituals, reflections, and reminders that help bring calm and focus back into everyday life.

It isn't about perfection or adding more tasks to your day. It's about noticing what already helps you feel steady — the morning light, a deep breath, a quiet moment of gratitude — and giving those things more space. If you'd like a few suggestions on how to move through these pages in a way that feels natural for you, there's a short 'How to Use This Guide' section that offers some gentle guidance — but feel free to explore in your own way, at your own pace.

However you choose to use this book, let it be flexible.

Pick a page, try a practice, or simply read when you need a nudge toward calm.

Every small act of awareness is a step toward a more centred, grounded you.

Before we begin, it helps to understand where these practices come from — and why they have a real effect on both body and mind. For centuries, people across the world used simple grounding, breathing, and energy-balancing rituals to restore focus and wellbeing long before modern science explained why they worked. Today, research shows that these natural methods still support how our nervous system, energy, and overall balance respond to the world around us.

A Gentle Realisation

Sometimes we don't even notice how certain past experiences continue to influence how we think, feel, and react in life. Not because we haven't "moved on," but because our mind and body are beautifully designed to protect us from ever feeling the same pain again.

When something hurts deeply, it can quietly shape our patterns without us realising. It may show up as:

- guarding our heart
- expecting disappointment
- replaying old memories
- holding tension in our body
- wanting justice or closure
- avoiding certain situations or people

This doesn't mean we are broken or stuck.
It simply means a part of us is still trying to stay safe.

And when emotional tension remains inside us, the

body will often try to carry it.
Sometimes it shows up as tight shoulders, a heavy chest, headaches, disrupted sleep, stomach discomfort, fatigue, or a feeling of constant alertness.

Not as punishment — but as a gentle message:
"Something inside me needs my care." 🌙

✨ Affirmation:

"I am ready to release what no longer protects me."

When hurt is still active, holding on can feel like strength — like protection, like fairness, like staying in control.
And letting go can feel like risk — like losing power, or allowing what happened to be "okay."

But healing isn't about pretending it didn't matter.
And it isn't about forgiving before you're ready.

Healing is the moment you gently choose your

peace over the story that caused your pain.

Revenge feeds the wound. Healing closes it.
And only one of those paths gives you your life back.

With compassion, not force.
With intention, not pressure.
With kindness, not perfection.

This journey is not about forgetting.

It's about finally remembering yourself.

...You've got this. ✨

🌍 Ancient Wisdom & Energy Science

Long before modern research confirmed the link between nature and wellbeing, ancient cultures already understood it. They spent time outdoors, worked with natural materials, and lived in rhythm with the seasons. Without calling it "grounding" or "energy balance," they instinctively knew that being in direct contact with the earth helped calm the body and clear the mind.

Today, science gives us language for what they felt. The surface of the Earth carries a subtle negative electrical charge. When we walk barefoot on grass, sand, or soil, or when we touch natural materials, those negative ions flow into the body. They help to neutralise the excess positive charge that builds up from stress, pollution, and constant exposure to electronic devices. This simple exchange supports the body's ability to restore balance — both physically and emotionally.

Breathing plays an equally important role. Deep,

steady breathing increases oxygen in the bloodstream, lowers stress hormones, and activates the parasympathetic nervous system — the part of the body responsible for rest and recovery. Combined with grounding, it creates a complete reset for both body and mind.

Reconnecting with these natural elements isn't about adding something new to your life — it's about returning to what your body already understands. As you move through the practices ahead, you'll notice that every step, breath, and mindful pause draws on this same ancient wisdom, supported now by modern energy science.

And so, we start where every journey of balance begins — with bare feet, steady breath, and the quiet support of the Earth.

🌿 Part One – The Space Around You

Creating environments that breathe calm and clarity

We begin our journey with the spaces that hold us — the rooms, corners, and quiet places where we spend our days. Every object, scent, and colour around us carries energy; the way we arrange them can either scatter our focus or bring us back home to ourselves.

When life feels unsettled, our outer environment often mirrors that inner chaos. By gently tending to the spaces we inhabit, we send a signal to the mind and body that peace is possible — that order and calm can return. Cleansing, organising, and surrounding ourselves with living elements like plants and natural light are not superficial acts; they are quiet declarations of self-respect.

This part of the book invites you to rediscover your surroundings as allies in your healing process. Whether it's lighting a candle with intention, refreshing the air with sage, or simply letting sunlight in after a long night, each act becomes a reminder that peace is built one small choice at a time.

> "When your space breathes, so do you."

🌿 The Foot Bath for Grounding & Release

At the end of a long day, there's something ancient and reassuring about placing your feet in warm water. It's a small gesture, yet it carries the weight of surrender — a letting go of everything the world has asked of you.

Our feet are our roots; they carry us through every experience and silently absorb the energy of our journey. Taking time to cleanse and comfort them is more than physical care — it's a ritual of grounding, connection, and release.

A foot bath reminds us that healing doesn't have to be grand. It lives in the smallest acts of kindness we offer ourselves.

You'll Need:

- A bowl or basin of warm water

- A handful of sea salt or Epsom salt

- A few drops of essential oil — lemon for renewal, eucalyptus for clarity, or lavender for calm

- A towel and a quiet moment to yourself

How to Begin:

1. Find a comfortable place to sit and rest your feet in the warm water.

2. As the salt dissolves, set your intention:

"With this water, I release what no longer serves me."

3. Close your eyes and take slow breaths, imagining the warmth drawing tension out through your soles.

4. When you're ready, lift your feet, pat them dry, and thank them for carrying you through another day.

Reflection Prompt:

- What am I ready to let go of, and what new energy would I like to welcome in its place?

🌿 Grounding — Returning to the Earth

In today's world, many people live more in their thoughts than in their bodies. We think, analyse, plan, worry, predict, compare, scroll and react — often without noticing how disconnected we have become from the physical world beneath us. Life has shifted from experiencing to processing, and while our minds have adapted to constant stimulation, our nervous systems have not. Grounding, sometimes called "earthing", is a way of returning to the present moment by reconnecting with physical reality — our bodies, our senses, and the natural environment we belong to.

The idea of grounding is not new. Long before technology, cities, office buildings and digital demands, humans instinctively lived close to the earth. They walked barefoot, slept on natural surfaces, spent most of their time outside, and observed nature not as an escape, but as part of everyday life. Their wellbeing was automatically supported by the environment they were immersed in. Today, we spend most of our hours indoors, surrounded by artificial light, electromagnetic devices, synthetic materials and over-stimulating noise, with very little direct contact to nature. Our bodies feel this absence, even if our minds do not immediately recognise it.

From a biological and neurological perspective, grounding has a calming effect because it activates the parasympathetic nervous system, often referred to as the rest and restore mode. This is the opposite of the fight, flight or freeze response. When we ground ourselves — whether through breath, touch, nature, or focused awareness — we send a clear message to the brain that we are safe. When the brain senses safety, stress hormones reduce, muscles release tension, breathing becomes steadier, and thinking becomes clearer. We are no longer operating from instinct or fear, but from balance and awareness.

Many ancient cultures understood grounding naturally, without needing scientific language. They practiced slow breathing, meditation, walking barefoot, sitting by firelight, bathing in natural waters, holding stones or wood for comfort, and spending long periods outside. These practices were not labelled as "therapies" or "techniques" — they were simply part of being human. Today, science provides explanations for what they already knew: the body works better when it feels connected, supported and safe.

Modern research shows that grounding can help reduce stress, support emotional regulation, improve focus, stabilise mood, and increase feelings of clarity and inner peace. It is not about changing who we are — it is about returning to who we always were, beneath the noise of daily life. Grounding reminds us that we are not only thinkers; we are breathing, sensing, feeling beings with physical needs that technology cannot replace.

There are many ways to ground, and each person may naturally be drawn to different methods. Some feel most rooted indoors through stillness and breathwork, while others require connection with nature to experience the same effect. The important thing is not how you ground, but that you do.

When practiced regularly, grounding becomes more than a technique — it becomes a personal reset, a way of returning to the body and the present moment before stress takes over.

In the following pages of this book, you will discover simple, practical grounding techniques that require no equipment, no expertise and no complicated preparation. They are gentle, accessible and adaptable to any lifestyle. If you approach them with openness and curiosity, you may find that grounding becomes not only a calming tool, but a supportive habit that strengthens your wellbeing long-term.

Grounding does not promise perfection, nor does it remove life's challenges. Instead, it gives you the internal stability to face life with clarity rather than overwhelm. Each time you ground, you take one small step back into balance — and with practice, that step becomes natural rather than forced.

Modern Reality: The Battery

Think of your mind and body like a device running on limited battery power. Every thought you overanalyse, every worry you carry, every decision you rush, and every problem you try to mentally solve drains a small percentage of that power. Before long, you may find yourself running on low energy without understanding why — not because you are weak, but because you are disconnected from your power source.

Grounding is the human equivalent of plugging yourself back in. It is not a quick boost like caffeine or distraction, but a steady recharge that restores clarity, balance, and inner strength. Without it, you may continue functioning, but everything feels heavier, slower, and more overwhelming than it needs to be.

Nature's Mirror: The Tree

Just like a tree cannot grow stronger by forcing its branches higher into the sky, neither can we grow by living only inside our thoughts. A tree becomes stable by deepening its roots into the earth, where it finds nourishment, support, and safety.

Grounding offers us the same foundation. It is not about achieving more or reaching further, but about returning to what sustains us. When we are rooted, growth becomes natural rather than forced, and life feels more like unfolding rather than struggling.

Whether you relate more to batteries or trees, the message is the same — life becomes easier when you are connected to what supports you.

When grounding becomes familiar within the body, our attention gently rises outward — to the rooms, objects, and atmospheres we live among. Here begins the quiet art of shaping our surroundings into spaces that feel safe, calm, and quietly alive.

🌿 Seasonal Energy — Living in Flow with Nature

A tree never apologises for shedding its leaves.
The butterfly doesn't rush its cocoon.
Every living being follows its own quiet rhythm of becoming — growth, stillness, renewal.
We are no different.

Just as the earth moves through her cycles of growth, harvest, rest, and rebirth, we too have seasons of expansion and retreat.

When we learn to move with these natural rhythms, we stop chasing the next moment and begin to inhabit this one.
Nature exists only in the present — it doesn't hurry toward spring or cling to summer.

By grounding ourselves in the here and now, we soften the anxious pull of "what's next" and rediscover calm in simply being.

Living in flow with the seasons allows our energy, mood, and self-care to align with the quiet wisdom of nature herself.

You'll Need

- Awareness of your surroundings — what's blooming, what's fading, what's shifting

- Willingness to slow down and listen to your body's seasonal cues

- A journal or planner to note reflections or intentions each season

How to Begin

1. Notice the transitions.

Step outside and truly observe — the scent in the air, the light, the colour of the leaves or sky. Let nature show you what's changing.

2. Reflect your rhythm.

Tune in to how your energy mirrors the season:

- 🌱 Spring — renewal, ideas, planting intentions

- ☀ Summer — expression, action, connection

- 🍂 Autumn — release, reflection, gratitude

- ❄ Winter — rest, restoration, inner stillness

3. Align your rituals.

- In spring, set new goals and cleanse your space.

- In summer, expand socially and move your body more freely.

- In autumn, focus on letting go — declutter, journal, prepare for quiet.

- In winter, rest deeply, nourish your body, and reflect.

4. Honour your internal seasons.

   Even when the calendar says "summer," your soul might be in "autumn." Follow your inner cues a above all else.

5. Celebrate the cycle.

   Mark each season's arrival with a small ritual — a candle, a walk in nature, or a note of gratitude to the earth.

Reflection Prompt

- What season of life am I in right now, and how can I support myself in this phase rather than resist it?

🌀 Alternative Ways to Try

If getting outdoors isn't always possible:

🌿 Bring the season inside – decorate with natural colours or textures that mirror the world outside.

🕯️ Shift your lighting – brighter in spring and summer, softer and warmer in autumn and winter.

🎶 Tune into sound – play music that reflects the mood of each season.

💜 Accessibility note:

Even if you can't physically be in nature, you can still attune to it — through imagery, scent, sound, and intention. Nature's rhythm lives within you too.

✦ **Affirmation**

"I move with the rhythm of nature.
In every season, I am renewed."

🌿 A Breath of Fresh Air — For You and Your Home

We often forget that the air around us affects our body just as much as the food we eat.

Fresh air carries oxygen — the fuel your cells, lungs, and nervous system rely on to reset, repair, and restore balance.

When a room stays closed for too long, the air becomes heavy with moisture from everyday breathing, cooking, and living.

This stale air can make the space feel dense, affect your sleep, and even make it harder to regulate temperature.

A short burst of fresh air — even for just a few minutes a day — helps:

- bring oxygen back into your space

- support clearer thinking and deeper breathing

- reduce trapped moisture

- create a lighter, more energising environment

Think of it as "ventilating your energy."

A reset for you, and for the home that holds you.

🌿 Cleansing with Sage & Sacred Smoke

There is an ancient comfort in watching smoke rise and dissolve into the air. Across cultures, the act of burning herbs or resins has always been a way of marking transition — of clearing what has been and making space for what's next.

Cleansing with smoke isn't about banishing "bad" energy as much as it is about setting intention. It's an act of mindfulness: the slow strike of the match, the soft curl of smoke, the breath you take as you move through the room.

With every gentle wave of your hand, you're reminding yourself that you have agency over what you allow into your space and your heart.
You don't have to use sage specifically; cedar, rosemary, lavender, or incense can all serve the same purpose. What matters is your focus and respect for the ritual.

You'll Need:

- A bundle of dried sage or your chosen cleansing herb

- A fireproof dish or shell

- Matches or a lighter

- (Optional) a small window open to let the old energy drift away

How to Begin:

1. Take a moment to centre yourself. Feel your feet on the floor.

2. Light the end of the bundle until it catches, then gently blow out the flame, letting the embers glow.

3. Move slowly around your space, guiding the

smoke into corners, around doorways, and over objects you use often.

4. As you do, repeat a quiet intention such as:

> "May this home hold peace, clarity, and light."

5. When you finish, extinguish the bundle safely and take a moment to feel the stillness that follows.

Reflection Prompt:

- What am I ready to release from this space, and what feeling would I like to invite in its place?

🌿 The Power of Salt Lamps & Real Plants

When the air feels heavy or the days begin to blur together, small, living anchors can quietly bring you back to centre. Nature is never far from us — even within four walls, we can invite its rhythm and purity into our homes.

Salt lamps and real plants are more than decorations; they are steady companions that cleanse, balance, and breathe with us. A salt lamp emits a soft, amber glow that mimics the gentleness of dawn. Its light is grounding, especially in the evening when screens and fluorescent bulbs overstimulate the senses.

Placed on a bedside table, desk, or meditation corner, it acts as a beacon of calm — a reminder to slow your breath and soften your gaze.
Plants, on the other hand, embody life itself. Their quiet persistence mirrors our own resilience; they

transform stale air, add moisture, and offer colour when the world feels grey. Tending to them — watering, pruning, repositioning — becomes a small meditation in care and presence.

You'll Need:

- A Himalayan salt lamp or natural salt crystal light.

- One or two easy-to-care-for plants (such as peace lilies, ferns, or spider plants)

- A clean, well-ventilated spot where light can reach.

How to Begin:

1. Place your salt lamp somewhere you'll often see it. Each evening, turn it on as the day winds down — let its glow signal the shift from doing to being.

2. Choose a plant that suits your space and lifestyle.
   As you care for it, imagine each drop of water or new leaf symbolising your own renewal.

3. Take a few quiet moments near your lamp and plant each day. Let yourself notice how the air feels fresher, the light warmer, your mood steadier.

Reflection Prompt:

- How does the energy of my space shift when I bring in elements that are alive and luminous?

🌿 Feng Shui Flow — Inviting Harmony into Your Home

Energy moves through a home the same way water moves through a stream. When its flow is blocked, we feel stagnant, heavy, and unsure of why. But when we create pathways for that energy to circulate freely, even the simplest rooms begin to feel lighter, more spacious, and alive.

Feng Shui — the ancient art of arranging space in harmony with natural forces — isn't about strict rules or superstition. It's about awareness: how your environment supports or drains you. It invites you to look at your surroundings with new eyes, noticing where energy pools and where it struggles to move.

A cluttered hallway might feel like a dam; a neglected corner can hold the weight of unspoken emotions. By gently shifting a few things — opening a window, repositioning a chair, adding a mirror to reflect light — you invite vitality back in.

This practice encourages you to listen to your intuition. If something feels off, it probably is. Let your inner sense of flow guide you as much as any diagram or compass.

You'll Need:

- A willingness to observe your space with honesty
- A clear intention (e.g., "I want my home to feel open and restful")
- Time to walk slowly through your home, noticing what draws or repels your energy

How to Begin:

1. Stand at your front door and take a deep breath. How does it feel to enter your home? Inviting? Heavy? Neutral?

2. Move through each room with curiosity. Notice cluttered areas, dark corners, or spots that don't feel comfortable.

3. Clear pathways so that energy can flow easily move furniture slightly, open curtains, add a plant or crystal where light needs to land.

4. Use scent and sound to refresh the air: a few drops of essential oil, gentle music, or the faint hum of wind chimes.

5. As you finish, pause to sense how the room now feels. Does your breath come easier? Do you feel more at ease? That's harmony beginning to return.

Reflection Prompt:

- What simple changes can I make today that will help my space — and my spirit — flow more freely?

🌿 Aromatherapy & Candles — Lighting Your Intention

Scent has a way of speaking directly to the soul. Long before words or reason, our bodies recognise it — the sharp freshness of lemon, the grounding earthiness of patchouli, the comfort of warm vanilla. A single breath can transport us to a memory or shift the rhythm of our thoughts.

Aromatherapy uses this quiet language to help us return to balance. When combined with candlelight, it becomes both a sensory experience and a symbolic one — fire for transformation, scent for mood, and light for presence. The simple act of lighting a candle can become a meditation, a way of saying: "I am here, and I am ready to begin again."

This practice invites you to create a small ritual of scent and flame to soothe or uplift your energy. It doesn't have to be elaborate; one candle and a mindful breath are often enough.

You'll Need:

- A candle (scented or plain)

- Optional: essential oils or an oil diffuser

- A safe, quiet spot where you can sit for a few minutes uninterrupted

How to Begin:

1. Before lighting your candle, take a moment to set an intention. It might be as simple as "peace," "focus," or "release."

2. If using oils, add a few drops to your diffuser or a bowl of warm water nearby.

3. Light the candle slowly, watching the flame flicker to life. Let its glow fill the room and soften your gaze.

4. As you breathe, let the scent and warmth

wrap gently around you. Imagine your intention taking shape in the air — calm, steady, luminous.

5. When you're ready, blow out the candle mindfully, as though sealing that intention into your heart.

Reflection Prompt:

- What emotion or energy do I wish to invite into my space today, and how does this scent remind me of it?

💧 Part Two – The Body You Live In

Supporting your physical energy and inner balance

Our bodies are the homes we carry everywhere. They hold our stories, our memories, our emotions — and just like any space, they thrive when tended to with gentleness and respect.

When life feels heavy, it's easy to forget that the body is always listening: to our thoughts, to the pace we move, to the nourishment we offer. By bringing awareness back into the body, we begin to reconnect with its quiet wisdom — that deep, wordless knowing that whispers, "I know how to heal."

This part of your journey is about tuning in, offering your body what it truly needs, and creating small, nurturing habits that build strength and serenity from the inside out.

> "When you care for the body,
> the soul feels seen."

💧 Hydration & Natural Detox

Water is the simplest medicine nature gives us, yet we often underestimate its quiet power. Every cell, every thought, and every emotion flows more freely when we are hydrated. It's not just about drinking enough — it's about honouring water as the element that carries energy through us, cleansing and renewing as it moves.

When we consciously hydrate, we're reminding ourselves to let go and begin again. The body releases tension more easily; the mind feels clearer. Adding small rituals around drinking water — a squeeze of lemon in the morning, a favourite glass kept nearby, a mindful pause between sips — transforms a routine into an act of self-respect.

You'll Need:

- A glass or bottle of water

- Optional: a slice of lemon, cucumber, or a few mint leaves

- A quiet moment to reconnect with your breath

How to Begin:

1. Before your first sip, take a deep breath. Feel gratitude for the water and what it brings.

2. As you drink, imagine each swallow carrying freshness and clarity through your system.

3. Throughout the day, keep water within reach. Let it be a gentle reminder to slow down, to refresh, to flow.

4. Once a week, if it feels right, support your body's natural detox by choosing lighter meals and staying hydrated — think herbal teas, soups, fruits, and greens.

Reflection Prompt:

- What does my body feel like when I listen to its needs instead of rushing past them?

💧 Vitamins, Minerals & B12 — Nourishment for Cyclical Balance

Our bodies are remarkable storytellers. They whisper their needs through cravings, fatigue, mood shifts, or changes in our rhythm — especially for those who experience hormonal cycles. When we begin to listen instead of override, nourishment becomes an act of partnership rather than control.

Vitamins and minerals are the body's quiet allies. They don't shout; they sustain. B12, magnesium, and iron, for instance, are the unsung heroes of balance — supporting energy, mood stability, and menstrual harmony. When these are low, the world can feel heavier, emotions sharper, and clarity harder to reach. But when we replenish what's been depleted, our vitality returns like sunlight breaking through clouds.

Food is information as much as fuel. Each meal can become a message of love to your body: I see you. I hear you. I will nourish you.

You'll Need:

- Foods rich in natural vitamins and minerals — leafy greens, nuts, seeds, colourful fruits, and whole grains

- If plant-based, consider adding B12 supplementation or fortified foods

- Gentle curiosity about what your body truly needs (and not what trends dictate)

How to Begin:

1. Start by noticing how you feel after you eat certain meals — energised, tired, calm, bloated, clear? Your body's feedback is instant wisdom.

2. Add one nutrient-rich habit each week — a green smoothie, magnesium-rich almonds, or iron-supporting lentils.

3. If you menstruate, track your cycle and notice where energy dips. Support those days with extra hydration, warm foods, and rest.

4. Approach food as medicine, but also as pleasure — balance nourishment with joy.

Reflection Prompt:

- What does balanced nourishment feel like in my body — lightness, clarity, steadiness, or ease?

💧 Reflexology — Touchpoints for Calm

Our hands and feet are quiet maps of the body — pathways of energy that connect to every organ, muscle, and emotion. When life feels overwhelming, a few minutes of intentional touch can bring us back into balance, reminding us that healing begins right where we are.

Reflexology isn't complicated; it's a language of care. By gently pressing or massaging specific points on the feet or hands, we stimulate the body's natural rhythms — supporting circulation, calming the nervous system, and easing tension that words can't reach. It's a practice of grounding, of coming home to yourself through the simplest form of connection: touch.

You don't need to know every reflex point to benefit. What matters most is awareness and intention — the way your breath slows, your shoulders drop, and you remember that your body and spirit are not separate.

You'll Need:

- Clean hands and a quiet moment

- Optional: a little oil or lotion

- A willingness to slow down and listen to your body's cues

How to Begin:

1. Sit comfortably and take a few deep breaths. Feel the weight of your body supported by the chair or floor.

2. Choose either your hands or feet. Apply a small amount of oil or lotion if you wish.

3. Using your thumb, apply gentle circular pressure to the soles of your feet or the palms

of your hands. Move slowly, noticing tender spots or areas that feel "stuck."

4. As you work, breathe into those areas, imagining light moving through them — clearing, soothing, restoring.

5. Finish by holding your hands or feet still for a moment, simply feeling warmth spread.

Reflection Prompt:

- What does my body ask for when I take the time to listen through touch rather than thought?

💧 Gentle Self-Massage & Body Awareness

The body speaks in sensation — tightness, warmth, fluttering, stillness. Yet so often we move through our days disconnected from those subtle messages. Gentle self-massage invites you back into conversation with your body, not to fix or change it, but simply to listen.

This is not about deep pressure or perfect technique. It's about presence. The simple act of placing your hands on your shoulders, neck, or legs with compassion tells your nervous system: You're safe. You can rest now. It reminds you that your body is not a machine to be managed, but a living, breathing ally in your healing.

When we touch ourselves with kindness, stress softens, emotions loosen, and awareness deepens. It's a return to trust — a quiet moment of reconciliation between body and soul.

You'll Need:

- A calm space where you won't be interrupted

- A few drops of your favourite oil or lotion (optional)

- A towel, cushion, or blanket for comfort

How to Begin:

1. Sit or lie comfortably and take three slow breaths.

2. Warm a little oil between your palms. Start with the shoulders or neck — wherever tension lingers.

3. Use slow, rhythmic strokes. Feel the texture of your skin, the temperature beneath your hands, the subtle shifts in breath and heartbeat.

4. Move to the arms, legs, or feet. Let the motion be intuitive rather than structured.

5. When finished, place your hands over your heart or abdomen. Feel your pulse. Whisper a quiet thank-you to your body for carrying you through.

Reflection Prompt:

- What parts of my body have been asking for care, and how can I honour them with gentleness today?

💧 Sleep, Rest & the Art of Stillness

Rest is the medicine the modern world forgets. We chase productivity as though peace were a prize to be earned — yet it's rest that makes everything else possible. True rest is not just sleep; it's a deep exhale of the spirit, a surrender into the arms of stillness.

Our bodies are wired for rhythm — waking, moving, pausing, replenishing. When that rhythm is broken, we feel it in every layer of ourselves: body tightens, mind races, spirit frays. But when we create simple rituals around rest, we teach our nervous system that it's safe to soften.

Stillness is not laziness. It's a conscious act of care. It's where the body repairs, the mind clears, and the heart remembers what matters.

You'll Need:

- A calm, darkened space

- Optional: soft lighting, a warm blanket, or gentle background sounds (rain, waves, ambient music)

- Willingness to slow down

How to Begin:

1. As evening approaches, dim the lights and silence distractions.

2. Do something to signal the day's end — sip herbal tea, stretch gently, or light a candle.

3. When you lie down, take three long breaths, releasing the day with each exhale.

4. If thoughts come, let them drift by like clouds. You don't need to chase or fix them.

5. Before sleep, whisper a simple intention: "May my rest restore me."

Reflection Prompt:

- What does true rest feel like in my body, and how can I create space for more of it in my life?

🔥 Part Three – The Energy Within

Listening to the quiet forces that move beneath thought

Once the outer world is tended and the body has been heard, the next layer of healing begins in the unseen — the energy that hums softly beneath everything you feel. This is the realm of intuition, vibration, and subtle awareness.

Energy is the language of connection: between people, between body and spirit, between the seen and unseen. You've already experienced it — that instinctive sense of someone's mood before they speak, the calm you feel in nature, the warmth of a comforting space. These are all expressions of energy at work.

This part of your journey is about noticing those

currents, learning how to balance them, and trusting that you can shape how they move through you. When your energy is clear and flowing, life feels more aligned. Decisions come easier, emotions settle faster, and purpose begins to whisper through the noise.

> "The more still you become, the more clearly you feel the energy that has always been guiding you."

🔥 Crystals & Their Healing Frequencies

Crystals are earth's memory keepers — formed over millions of years, shaped by pressure, fire, and time. Each one carries a unique vibration that resonates with different aspects of our energy field.

Whether or not you think of them as "magical," their natural beauty and quiet presence can remind us to stay centred, grounded, and open.

When you hold a crystal, you're not asking it to do the work for you; you're inviting partnership. The crystal becomes a symbol, a focus point for intention.

You'll Need:

- A few crystals that you feel drawn to (clear quartz, amethyst, rose quartz, black tourmaline, or Citrine are wonderful to start)

- A small pouch, bowl, or tray to keep them together

- A clean cloth or bowl of salt for cleansing

How to Begin:

1. Choose one or two crystals that "call" to you — trust your intuition.

2. Cleanse them before use by placing them in sunlight, moonlight, or a bowl of salt overnight.

3. Hold one in your hand and set an intention:

   "May this stone remind me of clarity and balance."

4. Keep it somewhere you'll see it often — your desk, bedside, or pocket — as a touchstone back to your intention.

5. Notice how the presence of your crystals subtly shifts the mood of your space or your energy throughout the day.

Reflection Prompt:

- What qualities do I most wish to amplify in my life right now, and how can I embody them as clearly as a crystal reflects light?

🔥 Developing Intuitive Awareness

Intuition isn't a mystical gift that only a few possess; it's the quiet voice that lives inside everyone. It's that moment when you just know something — the pull to call a friend, the sense that you should take a different route home, the feeling of ease when something is right.

When life is noisy or we spend too much time in our heads, that voice becomes harder to hear. But when we slow down and listen, intuition becomes one of our greatest guides. It speaks in sensations, emotions, and subtle cues from the body. The more we practice noticing, the clearer it becomes.

This practice isn't about predicting the future — it's about deepening trust in yourself. The goal is not to be "right" all the time, but to feel aligned with your own inner compass.

You'll Need:

- A quiet space for reflection

- A journal or notepad

- Optional: a small object for focus (a stone, candle flame, or even a pendulum if it feels right)

How to Begin:

1. Sit comfortably and take a few breaths to centre yourself.

2. Ask a simple question, such as "What do I need most today?" or "What will bring me peace right now?"

3. Notice the first impression that arises — not the loud thoughts that follow, but the subtle feeling underneath.

4. Write down what you sense without judging it. Over time, patterns will emerge and your confidence will grow.

5. For physical awareness, place a hand on your heart or belly and notice how your body feels when something is a clear "yes" versus a gentle "no."

Reflection Prompt:

- How does my intuition speak to me — through sensation, emotion, words, or knowing — and how can I make more space to listen?

🔥 Chakra Balancing & Cleansing Meditation

Your chakras are the body's subtle energy centres — seven spirals of light that move from the base of your spine to the crown of your head.

When they flow freely, you feel balanced, creative, confident, and calm.

When they're blocked, energy stagnates — you might feel heavy, uncertain, or emotionally clouded.

This meditation helps you reconnect, align, and gently clear those energetic pathways, bringing harmony back to your inner world.

You'll Need

- A quiet space where you can sit or lie comfortably

- Soft background music, a candle, or essential oils (optional)

- Your open heart and intention to restore balance

How to Begin

1. Sit or lie down comfortably. Close your eyes and take a slow, deep breath in through the nose and out through the mouth.

2. Visualise a warm, golden light entering the top of your head. As you breathe, let it travel down through each chakra, pausing briefly at each one.

3. With each breath, imagine the light gently clearing old energy — fear, doubt, tension — and replacing it with calm, vibrant flow.

If you're new to chakra work, use this simple guide:

🌸 Root (Base of Spine) – red light – Safety, grounding, stability

- ♥ Sacral (Below Navel) – orange light – Creativity, pleasure, flow

- ♥ Solar Plexus (Stomach) – yellow light – Confidence, strength, purpose

- ♥ Heart (Centre of Chest) – green or pink light – Love, compassion, connection

- ♥ Throat (Throat Area) – blue light – Expression, truth, voice

- ♥ Third Eye (Between Eyebrows) – indigo light – Intuition, clarity, insight

- ♡ Crown (Top of Head) – violet or white light – Spiritual connection, peace, unity

4. Spend a few breaths with each chakra, envisioning it glowing brighter and clearer with every inhale.

5. When you reach the crown, visualise all seven lights glowing together — a radiant column of energy connecting earth and sky.

6. Whisper a gentle affirmation of alignment:

"I am balanced, centred, and whole."

Reflection Prompt

- Which chakra felt most active or tender today? What message might that part of me be trying to share?

🌀 Alternative Ways to Try

If sitting still for meditation isn't ideal, you can still balance your energy:

💃 Movement meditation – sway or stretch slowly, imagining each motion clearing a different chakra.

🎨 Colour therapy – wear or surround yourself with colours linked to the chakras that feel out of balance.

🎵 Sound healing – listen to frequencies, chants, or singing bowls tuned to each chakra tone.

💜 Accessibility note:

Energy flows through intention more than position. Whether lying down, seated, or visualising from your bed — your energy still listens.

✨ **Affirmation**

"Light flows freely through me. I am aligned, open, and connected to all that is."

🔥 Journaling as Energy Release

There is a quiet alchemy that happens when ink meets paper.

What once lived silently inside you — thoughts, emotions, echoes of old stories — finds a voice.

Through journaling, energy begins to move. What felt heavy softens; what felt tangled slowly unravels.

You'll Need

- A journal that feels like an old friend, or even a single sheet of paper

- A pen that flows easily, allowing your words to follow their own rhythm

- A small pocket of stillness — perhaps a candle, soft light, or gentle music if you wish

How to Begin

1. Close your eyes and take three deep breaths. Let the exhale clear a little space inside.

2. Whisper an intention:

    "I release what no longer serves me. I write to understand, not to perfect."

3. Let your hand move across the page without editing or judging. Trust what arrives.

If you're unsure where to start, let these simple prompts open the door:

- "Today I'm holding onto…"
- "I'm proud of myself for…"
- "Right now, I need more…"
- "I forgive myself for…"

4. Pause now and then to feel your body — your heart rate, your breath, the easing of your shoulders.

5. When you finish, read only if it feels nurturing. Sometimes the writing itself is the release.

6. End with gratitude: for your honesty, your courage, and your willingness to show up.

Reflection Prompt

- What shifted within me as I gave my thoughts a voice? What truth surfaced between the lines?

🌀 Alternative Ways to Try

If writing isn't calling to you today, expression can take other shapes:

🎙️ Speak your release – record a voice note or speak softly to yourself. Sound carries energy out of the body.

🎨 Create your release – sketch, paint, or collage what you feel. Colour is another language of the soul.

🍃 One line a day – a single sentence can hold an entire world of meaning.

💜 Remember:

This isn't about eloquence — it's about honesty. However you choose to express, your truth deserves space to breathe.

✦ **Affirmation**

- "Through every word I write, I return home to myself."

🌾 Part Four — Bringing It Together

This final part of your journey is about weaving everything you've learned into a life that feels steady, supported, and genuinely yours.
Not a perfect life — but a balanced one.

By now, you've tended to your surroundings, honoured your body, and explored the quiet language of your inner energy. Part Four brings these pieces together and grounds them into simple daily rhythms — the kind that create peace without forcing it, and alignment without pressure.

This is where wellness becomes a way of living rather than something you chase.

Here, you'll build gentle routines, reconnect with nature's seasons, carve out moments of calm, and create a personal resilience kit you can return to whenever life becomes loud.

This is where everything comes together —
into a version of you who moves with intention,
acts with clarity, and comes home to yourself again
and again.

Building Daily & Weekly Routines

Healing and growth rarely arrive in grand gestures — they live quietly in the rhythm of our days.

A mindful routine isn't about rules or rigidity; it's about creating small, sacred anchors that help your energy stay balanced when life moves fast.

Through consistency and compassion, even the simplest habits become rituals of alignment and care.

You'll Need

- A notebook or planner — digital or paper, whatever feels natural

- Awareness of your natural energy flow — morning, midday, and evening

- Gentle curiosity about what truly nourishes your body, mind, and spirit

How to Begin

1. Start small. Choose one or two nurturing practices from this guide — perhaps journaling, a short meditation, or mindful hydration — and weave them naturally into your day.

2. Create anchor moments.

    Morning: A breath of gratitude, setting a daily intention.

    Midday: A short walk, gentle stretch, or mindful pause.

    Evening: Reflection, journaling, or a Candlelit moment of calm.

3. Shape your weekly rhythm.

   Pick one restorative activity each week — a digital detox evening, a creative session, or a quiet nature walk.

   On Sundays, reflect gently: What supported me this week? What drained me? Adjust with kindness.

4. Stay flexible. Routines should serve you, not restrict you. Honour your natural cycles and allow space for both rest and flow.

5. Celebrate small consistencies. Transformation happens quietly. Every time you show up for yourself, you strengthen the foundation of your well-being.

Reflection Prompt

- Which moments in my day feel most like home? How can I honour them and build around them?

🌀 Alternative Ways to Try

If structure feels overwhelming, think in themes instead of fixed schedules:

- 🌿 Nurture Days — slow pace, comfort food, rest.
- ☀️ Flow Days — creativity, movement, connection.
- 🌙 Reset Moments — three deep breaths, a stretch, a quiet pause between tasks.

💜 Accessibility note:

A mindful routine is about intention, not perfection. Adapt your rhythm to your lifestyle, health, and energy — every gentle effort counts.

✨ Affirmation

> "Through gentle consistency, I become my own sanctuary."

🌙 Moments of Light — Daily Reflections for Calm

Peace isn't something we chase; it's something we notice.
Moments of calm already exist all around us — a breath, a beam of sunlight, the warmth of a cup in your hands.

When we learn to pause and witness these tiny moments of light, they become anchors — gentle reminders that serenity doesn't live in the future; it lives in the now.

These reflections help you reconnect with presence, gratitude, and the quiet beauty that often hides in plain sight.

You'll Need

- A few quiet minutes in your day

- A journal or notepad (optional)

- A willingness to slow down and let the world meet you where you are

How to Begin

1. Create a daily pause.

   Choose one or two moments each day — morning coffee, an evening walk, or even the commute home — to simply be.

2. Observe without expectation.

   Notice the sounds, textures, colours, or Sensations around you. Let yourself feel grounded in what is.

3. Reflect gently.

Ask yourself:

- What brought me a moment of peace today

- What beauty did I almost overlook?

- What am I grateful for right now?

4. Capture the light.

   Write down one sentence, phrase, or word that sums up your calm moment. Over time, these small notes become a mosaic of peace — proof that light is always present, even on quieter days.

5. End with a slow breath.

   Let gratitude soften your body and mind. The moment doesn't need to last forever to change how you feel.

Reflection Prompt

- Where did I find a moment of stillness today, and what did it teach me about slowing down?

✦ Affirmation

"I carry light within me – it never truly fades"

🌀 Alternative Ways to Try

If journaling isn't practical or appealing:

📷 Photo reflections — capture a single calming image each day, something that made you pause or smile.

🕯 Evening recall — before bed, replay one gentle moment from the day in your mind.

🎶 Sound reflections — notice soothing sounds around you — birdsong, rain, laughter — and take a deep breath to absorb their peace.

💜 Accessibility note:

Stillness doesn't always mean silence or solitude. Even in a busy space, one mindful breath can reconnect you to calm.

✨ **Affirmation**

"Peace lives in the present. I am here, and this moment is enough."

🌟 Gratitude, Faith & Trusting the Process

Gratitude is the language of trust.

It's how we tell life, "I see the good, even when I don't see the full picture."

When you practise gratitude, you shift from striving to receiving.

Faith grows in that same soil — the understanding that every delay, every detour, every quiet season carries its own purpose.

Trusting the process doesn't mean pretending everything is perfect; it means believing that each step, even the uncertain ones, is shaping you into who you are becoming.

You'll Need

- A few minutes at the beginning or end of each day

- A journal or simple notepad

- A willingness to look for light, even on the grey days

How to Begin

1. Start small.

   Each day, name three things you're grateful for. They don't have to be grand — a kind word, a warm meal, a moment of laughter all count.

2. Feel it.

   Take a breath after each one and feel the gratitude in your body. Let it land.

3. Reflect on timing.

   Think of something that once felt like a Setback but later revealed its purpose.

   - What did it teach you?

   - How did it prepare you for something better aligned?

4. Build faith.

   Write a small affirmation of trust:

   "I may not know how it all unfolds, but I trust that I'm being guided."

5. End in surrender.

   Light a candle or simply close your eyes and whisper thank you — not for the outcome, but for the journey.

Reflection Prompt

- Where in my life can I practise gratitude for what is, while trusting what's yet to come?

🌀 Alternative Ways to Try

If journaling doesn't fit your day:

💬 Spoken gratitude – say thank you aloud during your routine, like a soft prayer woven into your actions.

📷 Gratitude snapshots – take photos of little blessings through the week; revisit them when faith feels thin.

🕯 Quiet appreciation – pause at the end of the day, place your hand over your heart, and silently give thanks for the moments that kept you going.

💜 Accessibility note:

Gratitude doesn't require perfect conditions — it grows wherever it's planted. Even the smallest thanks creates space for peace.

✦ **Affirmation**

"I trust in divine timing. Every moment serves my becoming."

Your Personal Resilience Kit

"Resilience is not about being unshaken — but knowing where to return when you tremble."

The Five Pillars of Everyday Resilience

*

1) Awareness & Inner Noticing

> Resilience begins with recognising how you are, not judging it.
> This may include pausing before reacting, naming emotions without analysing, noticing tension or tiredness, or asking:
>
> *"What is my body telling me right now?"*
>
> Awareness is not weakness — it is the Doorway to change.

⋆

2) Emotional Soothing & Regulation

When emotions rise, the aim is not to suppress them, but to support your nervous system back into safety.

Helpful approaches may include grounding touch, slow breathing, warm comfort, gentle movement, or releasing thoughts through writing or voice notes.

Regulation says: *"I am allowed to feel — and I am able to settle."*

⋆

3) Energy & Environment Protection

Your surroundings and your boundaries

influence how you feel.

This may look like keeping one area calm, limiting draining conversations, protecting mornings or evenings, or allowing quiet time without apology.

You are not withdrawing — you are Choosing where your energy lives.

★

4) Body Support & Gentle Care

Resilience grows when the body feels supported and resourced.

Kind actions may include regular hydration, nourishing foods, movement that feels good, and sleep patterns that suit your personal rhythm.

Your body is not an obstacle — it is part of

your team.

*

5) Identity, Meaning & Forward Direction

You are not who you were before the challenging moments — you are becoming someone wiser.

Explore the values you now live by, and what peace means to you, and small steps that build self-trust.

You may ask:

"What would my future self-thank me for?"

Resilience develops through the decisions that support who you are becoming.

🌱 A Pocket Reminder

"I am allowed to move slowly.

I am allowed to protect my peace.
I am allowed to choose what supports the person I am becoming."

Personal Practice Page

My top three grounding supports:

1.
_____

2.
_____

3.
_____

When I need help, I will reach for:

_____

A message of encouragement to my future self:

_____

_____

_____

This kit is not a test — it is your gentle return point.
Come back to it anytime you need grounding, clarity, or a reminder that healing is not linear but always possible.

🌙 Leaving Work Behind & Coming Home to Yourself

A gentle transition ritual for the mind, body, and heart.

When you come home at the end of the day, your whole system deserves a moment to shift — from responsibility to rest, from doing to being, from thinking to feeling.

This chapter guides you through a simple sequence that helps you release the day and return to yourself with clarity, calm, and warmth.

1) The Doorway Chime Ritual

Marking the moment you step back into your life.
As you cross your front door, pause for just one second.
Gently ring your chime.

Let the sound travel ahead of you — soft, light, cleansing.

This is your signal:

"I'm home now."

The vibration helps your body release the workday before you even take another step inside. It sets the tone for everything that follows.

2) Grounding Exercises to Release Work Energy

Settling your body after the chime has cleared the air.

Once the sound fades, place your feet firmly on the floor.

Take a slow breath in… and an even slower breath out.

Feel your body shift from "alert" into "safe."

You can choose any grounding method you like:

🫁 The 4–6 breath

Inhale for 4

Exhale for 6

Repeat a few times.

👐 Hand-to-body grounding

Place one hand on your chest, one on your stomach.

Feel your body soften beneath your touch.

👣 Feet awareness

Notice the floor supporting you.

Let your weight sink gently into it.

Let your body know:

"You can relax. The day is over."

3) Protecting Your Home as a Sanctuary

Creating a peaceful space where work cannot follow.

Your home deserves to feel like a safe place again — not an extension of your workplace.

Before you move deeper into the house, imagine taking off an invisible "coat" filled with the stress of the day. When you remove your real coat, let the energy fall away with it.

Say quietly:

"What's outside stays outside."

Open a window if you like.
Light a candle.
Turn on soft music.
Let the space welcome you back.

Your home is not another shift.
Your home is where you return to yourself.

4) Emotional Unloading: Leaving the Day Behind

Giving yourself permission to put the weight down.

Sometimes what stays with us is not the tasks — it's the emotions around them.

Before you continue your evening, take a moment to "unload" anything you're still carrying:

- a frustration
- a worry
- a conversation
- an unfinished thought
- someone else's bad mood

You can write it down, say it out loud, or imagine placing it in a mental basket by the door.

Tell yourself:

"I don't need to carry this inside my evening."

You're not avoiding anything —

you're allowing your nervous system to rest.

5) The Three-Minute Evening Reset

A simple ritual to bring your whole system back into balance.

If you take just one thing from this chapter, let it be this.

Three minutes.
A softer night.
A calmer mind.

🌙 Minute 1 — Clear the Mind

Ask yourself:

"Is there anything from today that still needs my attention right now?"

If yes, write it down.

If no, breathe out and let it fall away.

🌿 Minute 2 — Release the Body

Breathe in for 4

Breathe out for 6

Three times.

Your system will immediately begin to unwind.

✨ Minute 3 — Reset Your Energy

Close your eyes and say:

"Today is complete. I return to myself now."

Visualise your energy gathering back into your chest like warm light.

Reflection — *A Gentle Prompt*

A moment of gentle awareness.

Take a breath and ask yourself:

"What does coming home to myself feel like in my body?"

There is no right answer — only your truth.

6) Closing Note: Returning Home to Yourself

No matter how long or demanding your day has been, you deserve to end it with tenderness.

Your home is your sanctuary — a place that holds you, restores you, and reminds you of who you are beneath the noise of the world.

You have the right to put the day down.

You have the right to rest.

You have the right to come back to yourself.

And tonight... you do.

The Light You Carry Forward

You've journeyed through awareness, release, reflection, and renewal — not by becoming someone new, but by remembering who you already are.

Healing isn't about proving your worth to the world. It's about reclaiming your peace from the noise of comparison.

You were never meant to walk another's path or measure your pace against someone else's. The rhythm of your growth is your own — unique, sacred, and perfectly timed.

When you stop seeking validation in outside eyes, you begin to see your reflection clearly again — whole, worthy, and radiant exactly as you are.

Self-care is not selfish; it is self-honouring. It is the quiet act of saying, "I matter too."

So as you step beyond these pages, carry this truth with you:

You are not behind. You are not too late. You are right on time for your own becoming.

- Keep choosing presence over pressure.

- Keep choosing faith over fear.

- Keep choosing love — always love, over comparison.

Because the light you've been searching for was never out there.

It's been within you all along — quietly waiting for you to remember.

✨ **Final Affirmations**

> *"I honour my journey. I trust the timing of my life.*
>
> *"I am enough, I am light, and I am free."*

"You've spent time learning how to reconnect with your body, space, and spirit.

Each breath, each pause, each quiet choice brings you closer to balance.

Remember, coming home to Yourself is not a destination – it's a way of being." 🌿

A Note For Your Heart

If you ever find yourself believing you are the only one who feels this way, please remember this: the human brain is wired for emotional learning, protection, and connection. Many people experience similar thoughts, fears, and emotional patterns — even if they never speak them aloud.

Struggling doesn't mean you are weak — it often means your nervous system is trying to protect you by slowing you down until it feels safe to move forward.

"Pause. Breathe. You are doing better than you think."

Healing is not something you do against the world, but within a human community that is far more similar than it appears on the surface."

"Together, we can make each other feel heard."

www.ingramcontent.com/pod-product-compliance
Lightning Source LLC
Chambersburg PA
CBHW052059070526
44584CB00017B/2246